GET READY FOR YOUR
White Coat

GET READY FOR YOUR
White Coat

A Doctor's Guide on Getting into the
Best Medical Schools

OLATOKUNBO M. FAMAKINWA, MD, MPH

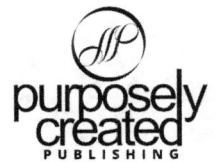

GET READY FOR YOUR WHITE COAT
Published by Purposely Created Publishing Group™
Copyright © 2018 Olatokunbo M. Famakinwa

All rights reserved.

No part of this book may be reproduced, distributed or transmitted in any form by any means, graphic, electronic, or mechanical, including photocopy, recording, taping, or by any information storage or retrieval system, without permission in writing from the publisher, except in the case of reprints in the context of reviews, quotes, or references.

Printed in the United States of America
ISBN: 978-1-949134-07-0

Doctor Toks's books and products are available through online book retailers. To contact DoctorToksMD.com directly, please email our Customer Service Department at

info@doctortoksmd.com.

LEGAL DISCLAIMER

Please note this book has not represented and does not provide any guarantee or warranty of any kind whatsoever, implied or otherwise, that the information provided in this book will improve anyone's chances for admission to postgraduate programs, BS/BA/MD programs, or medical school. By reading this book you acknowledge that the information is not to be construed as prophetic. Dr. Olatokunbo Famakinwa has no affiliation or relationship with any of the companies, organizations, or institutions mentioned in this book as of the time of writing.

The information in the book is not meant to be considered medical advice. Please always consult with your physician or licensed medical provider for medical attention. Patient names and all identifying information have been changed and/or omitted to protect patient privacy.

DEDICATION

It has been said that "the love of a family is life's greatest blessing." I will forever be grateful to God for such an amazing family. To my parents, Ola and Bukky: you both have sacrificed everything—including your own personal dreams—just for my success. I remember the days when Dad worked three jobs and Mom would work thirty-six hours straight so that I would have all of the things I needed (and sometimes, just so I wouldn't feel left out among my friends). To my siblings, Bisi, Sade and Kunle: you are the best siblings I could ever ask for—and continue to be the inspiration for everything that I do.

And of course, I must give special thanks to several of my closest friends—Senayet, Sabra, Jocelyn, Mariamawit, Victor, Chanel, Alexis, Christine, Tayo, Shantal, Ed, and Kamille—with whom I began the pre-med journey over fifteen years ago: thank you for standing by my side, for your encouraging words, for proofreading my (many) essays to get into medical school and beyond, and so much more. Your friendship is truly a gift.

TABLE OF CONTENTS

Introduction 1

Competence 7

Commitment to Medicine 27

Intellectual Curiosity 35

Compassion and Service 43

Teamwork and Communication 51

Ethical Principles and Integrity 59

Professionalism 67

Conclusion 73

References 77

About the Author 81

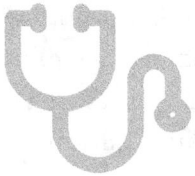

INTRODUCTION

I can imagine no greater privilege than to be a physician.

Yes, despite the thousands of hours spent studying, the difficult patient encounters, and the increasing complexity of our healthcare system—there is no greater calling than to be a doctor. To be trusted with the responsibility of caring for people at their weakest and most vulnerable moments is incredibly challenging, but also an immense honor. As you probably already know, becoming a doctor is no easy task. The journey begins with four years of college, during which you have to take several required courses in the sciences as well as mathematics. Then you have to go to medical school, which is another four years. This is all followed by a professional training period called residency. Residency can last anywhere from three to five years. After completing residency, you can finally practice as an independent physician. However, some doctors will choose to complete additional subspecialty training called a fellowship (think cardiology or critical-care medicine), which can take an average of an additional three years of training. Do the math—that's well over a decade spent pursuing a career in medicine. Talk about delayed gratification!

Let me share a little about my own journey. After graduating from Princeton University well over a decade ago (yikes!), I attended medical school at the Yale University School of Medicine. I stayed at Yale to complete a combined residency program in both internal medicine and pediatrics. I now work in hospital medicine, which I love. I am also passionate about helping others—I have personally advised hundreds of students on how to achieve their dreams of admission to top medical schools around the country. I spent nearly a decade in an advisory role for the Association of American Medical Colleges Summer Medical and Dental Education Program (SMDEP, a six-week summer experience for disadvantaged and underrepresented college students interested in medicine) at Yale University, and have also developed healthcare career programming for Yale undergraduates and young children in New Haven, Connecticut. Pursuing a medical career is quite a challenging endeavor and I feel so fortunate to have helped so many students in their quest.

While the road to becoming a physician is long, the most difficult step is actually getting into medical school. According to the Association of American Medical Colleges (AAMC), over 50,000 people applied to medical school in 2017—but only 21,338 students actually started medical school the following fall.[1] This means that only four out of ten people receive an acceptance letter in a given year. These statistics are pretty brutal.

So what makes a successful applicant? A quick Google search will likely bring up two answers: a high GPA and a great MCAT score. According to the AAMC, the average GPA of students who matriculated to medical school in 2018 was a 3.71, and the average score on the Medical College Admission Test (MCAT) score was a 510.4.[2] Indeed, the coursework in medical school is rigorous, and certainly your grades and test scores are useful tools to assess your academic potential and to predict your ability to handle the intense workload of a medical student.

But it is not just about your numbers.

Let's try a little exercise. Get on your computer or cell phone and go to the website of your favorite medical school. Do a quick search for the school's mission statement. Let's look at one of the top medical schools in the country, the University of North Carolina School of Medicine. The mission statement reads:

> Our mission is to improve the health and well-being of North Carolinians and others whom we serve. We accomplish this by providing leadership and excellence in the interrelated areas of patient care, education, and research.[3]

Try the same thing for University of Pittsburgh School of Medicine:

> To improve the health and well-being of individuals and populations through cutting-edge biomedical research, innovative educational programs in medicine and biomedical science, and leadership in academic medicine.[4]

And for what it's worth, you can also check out this bullet point from the mission statement of my alma mater, the Yale University School of Medicine:

> [to] educate and inspire scholars and future leaders who will advance the practice of medicine and the biomedical sciences.[5]

Do you notice a trend here? The mission of many medical schools—and especially the top medical schools—is to develop *leaders* in medicine. Becoming a leader in medicine is much more than scoring well on examinations and getting good grades. The reality is that medical schools could easily fill their entire class with people who have perfect GPAs and MCAT scores. Admissions committees are clearly looking for other characteristics—in addition to academic performance—when selecting future students.

That is where this guide comes in. To be clear, this is NOT an overview of the medical school admissions process itself. Frankly, the resources on admissions are endless, and the American Association of Osteopathic Schools and the AAMC both do an amazing job on their respective websites of explaining the dates and the details. My goal in writing this book is to touch upon the intangibles: the things that you can do, along with getting good grades and high test scores, to develop the skills and characteristics needed to be a leader in medicine. I want to provide you with a different framework as you start preparing to apply to medical school. I challenge you to refrain from thinking about the medical school admissions process as a "checklist" of tasks to complete. Rather, I hope this book will allow you to consider and understand the characteristics of what it takes to be a physician, as well as examine how such qualities align with your own values. The worst thing that can happen is for a person to spend so much time, and lots of money, trying to become a physician only to find that medicine is not for them. I have seen this happen too many times. This quick-read guide is designed to focus your approach while giving you a holistic perspective on what you need to be a doctor and leader in medicine. The sooner you understand the realities of pursuing a medical career, the better equipped you will be to craft your own journey and successfully navigate the process. Other books just tell you what to do. In this guide, I will not only tell you what to do, but also why you should do it.

This guide is organized as a review of seven key aspects of being a physician-leader: competence, commitment to medicine, intellectual curiosity, compassion and service, teamwork and communication, ethical principles, and professionalism. I will share my insights from the many lessons that I have learned personally over the years on my own journey in medicine, as well as from the experience of having worked with hundreds of students for nearly a decade. You will also occasionally see the "Keep It Real" box; this is where I will give honest (and sometimes tough!) answers to those common pre-med questions that you would rather not ask publicly. Hopefully, you will identify with some of my experiences (including my many fumbles!) as you think about your own journey toward becoming a physician.

I should probably take a moment here to mention my second motivation for writing this book. If you ask doctors who started to practice medicine twenty years ago about the state of medical practice today, they will likely share with you that the field has significantly changed. In many ways, the patient-doctor relationship is not at the center of medical practice. This shift has happened in part because doctors have been passive in advocating for patients and have allowed the financial interests of others to determine the direction of medical care. For this reason, I hope this book will help to inspire and motivate the next generation of medical professionals to be not just doctors, but also physician-leaders. Our field needs people who are willing to speak up and put the patient first.

Now, with that out of the way, let's do this.

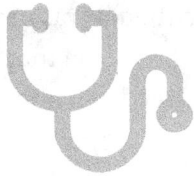

COMPETENCE

Decked in a pair of bleach-stained sweatpants and red flip-flops, I scaled the steep hill to find out my grade on my first college-level chemistry exam. Naturally, I was nervous. As I approached the building, the other students around me seemed so happy; they were smiling and laughing. This encouraged me and I began to think maybe this pre-med thing wasn't going to be so tough after all. That euphoria lasted only a few minutes; when I grabbed my exam and saw my grade my heart sank.

A big red F. I had failed.

I squinted my eyes in hopes that the harsh lines of the letter F would somehow magically change form. No, it was true, I had indeed failed. I was paralyzed for what seemed like an eternity.

I was absolutely mortified. I was used to doing well in high school, and this was the first time that I had ever struggled in a course. I had to take a step back and figure out where things went wrong. I definitely had spent a little too much time at the campus center "studying" with friends. My procrastination habits were never a problem for me in high school, but I clearly needed to change my approach if I wanted to get good grades in my freshman pre-med classes. After weeks of intense studying and spending a lot of time in office hours, I somehow passed the class. A miracle. I vowed to never let that happen again.

I managed to get an A- in my second semester of the course.

The reality of being a doctor is that you have to know your stuff. There is no getting around this.

Because of this, your pre-medical journey will start with taking classes that are the foundation of medical science. Students can make the mistake of assuming that there is a "pre-med" major in college, but such a major does not exist at most institutions. The term "pre-med track" is probably more appropriate, whereby you major in a course of study of your choice, but take a specific set of courses required for medical school admission. There may be slight variations between medical schools, but essentially these courses include a year of general chemistry, a year of organic chemistry, a year of biology, a semester of mathematics, and a year of physics. These courses make up what is called a BCPM (**B**iology, **C**hemistry, **P**hysics, and **M**athematics) GPA. Admissions committees pay special attention to this number. Because of this, as soon as you start your pre-medical journey you must map out your class schedule for the next three years. When will you have the time to fit in all of the required pre-med courses? It is critical to plan this out well in advance so that you take the pre-med courses at the time that works best for you. For example, if you are still an undergraduate student, you probably do not want to take organic chemistry, physics, and molecular biology in the same semester because the workload may be overwhelming and, in turn, may compromise your BCPM GPA. Additionally, try to complete most, if not all, of your pre-med courses before you take the MCAT, as these courses are the foundation of knowledge that you will need for the exam. If you do not have a clear plan for your coursework, it will take you much longer to actually start the application process to medical school.

Even if you are unclear about your plan for completing these required courses, don't fret—you can still get back on track. For example, you can take classes in the summer at another institution. This is not at all uncommon; I ended up taking physics during the summer at a nearby university. If you do need to take courses elsewhere, it is important that you attend a school that is at least similar in quality and standing to your undergraduate institution. I would recommend against taking any of the required pre-med classes at a community college. This is a harsh truth, but the reality is that many admissions professionals perceive the rigor and intensity of coursework at a community college less favorably than that of a four-year institution. Because of this perception, taking courses at a community college may give the impression to some that you are taking the "easy way" out. Remember, admissions committees not only consider the type of classes that you take, but also look to see that you have challenged yourself in your coursework.

Many pre-medical students make the mistake of choosing a science major because they think this is required in order to apply to medical school. This is just not true! Pursuing a science major may allow you to more easily complete the prerequisite courses for medical school, since many of the classes required for the major will overlap with the pre-med courses that are necessary to apply. However, you do not have to be a science major to get into medical school. Let me repeat that—you do NOT need to be a biology, chemistry, physics, or other science major to get into medical school!

You should major in a field of study that you are passionate about and, quite frankly, that you will do well in. For me, I have always loved history, so I became a history major while in college. I am not alone; a quick review of the most recent statistics from the AAMC demonstrates that there were over

3,000 students who majored in the humanities and social sciences that were accepted into medical school in 2017.[6]

Here is the caveat—if you do decide to major in a non-science field, make sure to do well in your BCPM courses. This is where I see students making big mistakes; they choose a non-science major AND do not perform well in their science classes. This raises a red flag for admissions officers, as a poor performance in the sciences may indicate that the student is not ready for the academic rigor of medical school. Additionally, if you have chosen to be a non-science major, be prepared to explain your decision—it will almost certainly come up later during the medical school interview process. Saying to an admissions director that you chose sociology because you thought it was easier than dealing with biochemistry is NOT the right answer to give during your interview. You should have a sensible reason and a clear thought process behind why you chose that particular major. Personally, I chose to major in history because I had a strong interest in how scientific knowledge has been created over the years and how social, political, and economic events influence the development of this knowledge.

We spent the last few pages reviewing what you need to do well. Now let's discuss how, practically, to make that happen. Having worked with students across a wide range of academic ability, here are seven basic guidelines that you can use to do well in your pre-med courses:

1. **Go to class.** This may seem obvious, but I have had so many students complain to me about getting bad grades—and on further questioning I discover that they never actually went to class. I often hear excuses like "the professor is terrible" or "I don't find class useful." While the quality of the classroom instruction may indeed vary, it is still always good practice to show up to class. If nothing else, this is the time when the professor can get to know your face, and it may even provide the opportunity for you to obtain a letter of recommendation in the future. If the material of the class comes easily to you, you can use your class time to demonstrate your interest and mastery of the material—but be sure to do so without coming across as obnoxious. Showing up to class will also give you the confidence to know that you didn't miss any important course material, which will in turn translate to the confidence that you need when it comes time for the final exam.

2. **Review the course syllabus.** As you go through the class, continuously reference the course syllabus to ensure that you are keeping up with all of the class requirements and are meeting the academic objectives. Make sure you understand what your professor will be testing on the exam, as well as the format of the examinations. The course syllabus will also show the deadlines for exams and papers so that you can plan ahead and determine when you need to start writing and studying.

3. **Start studying for the class on day one.** Every day, you should do a little bit to study for class. Do not wait until the last minute and hope that cramming the material will save you. It will not. In high school it is much easier to cram the material the night before, but college is a different beast all together. Put your best foot forward and avoid cramming.

4. **Find a study partner.** One of the biggest mistakes that students make is to study alone. In high school studying with others may not have been necessary, but having a study partner in college is a good idea because you have someone who will hold you accountable and hopefully inspire you during the tough times. You don't have to study with someone every single day, but either once a week or once every two weeks is helpful for additional review. Studying with others also provides you the opportunity to explain and teach the concepts that you are studying. A critical part of training as a physician is to teach others (both your patients AND your colleagues), so you will get great practice if you start now with a study buddy. Now, it is important to be honest with yourself; if your study partner is a distraction, you need to find a new study partner.

5. **Create a study routine and stick to it.** Before your classes start, it is worth scoping out the campus and

local coffee shops to see where you will have the best study environment. Does the place have good lighting? Is it crowded? Are the chairs comfortable? Are there bathrooms nearby? Choose your study space carefully; it will be your go-to location for the entire semester (if not longer). Also consider at what time of the day you study best. Are you a morning person? Then study before class. Night owl? Then get ready to burn the midnight oil. Create a schedule of when you will study and stick to it. Your time to study is just like having to go to a class. Another helpful tip: if you find yourself in transit for several hours a day, put your study materials on your smart phone and listen to lectures. Disconnect from social media apps if you need to in order to avoid distractions.

6. **Sleep.** Another overlooked aspect of creating a study routine is incorporating a good sleep routine! I cannot overemphasize the importance of a good sleep regimen. Good quality sleep makes you more attentive and helps with memory.

7. **Do not cram the night before the exam.** I must come back to this tip again. As tempting as it may be—and as busy as you may be—it is very important to avoid cramming the night before the exam. While cramming may work for some people, in the long run it is typically not beneficial. Remember that your sci-

ence courses are the foundation of the material on the MCAT exam. If you cram, you will likely have a weak knowledge base that may compromise your eventual performance on the MCAT. And let's face it, cramming is painful. I had many nights in college where I stayed up for over thirty-six hours in order to get in enough studying for an exam. And after taking the exam I always hated myself the next day (and usually ended up sick somehow in the student health center). Don't be like me. Save your nights of no sleep for when you are scheduled for 28 hour on-call shifts in the hospital.

KEEP IT REAL DR. TOKS:

Does it matter where I go to college?

Where you go to college is important, but it should not stop your dream of becoming a physician.

Many students ask this question, believing that if their college is not prestigious enough it will put them at a disadvantage during the admissions process. My answer?

The bottom line is, no matter where you go, you must do well.

1. Always go to the best college that you can. BE SURE to make the effort to do well—that's where being strategic from the start comes in.

2. If you go to a school that is less competitive, again, you must make every effort to do well. You need to show the admissions committee that you are capable of handling the intensity of learning in medical school.

If you have done well at a smaller, lesser-known, or less competitive school, this *may* actually weigh in your favor. A top-ranked school may have hundreds of students applying to medical school each year. But if you go to a small college that has only a few students applying to medical school each year, you may actually be a bit more memorable. You will stand out because you are not from an institution that admissions committees usually see.

Because of finances, family, and other obligations, you can't always control where you go to school. But you can control how well you do.

Let's talk a bit more about the MCAT. Having to take the MCAT is probably one of the most difficult parts of the admissions process to medical school. The MCAT exam assesses your knowledge of foundational principles in the natural, biological, and social sciences. The exam also evaluates your ability to think critically. The MCAT is made up of four sections: Chemical and Physical Foundations of Biological Systems, Biological and Biochemical Foundations of Living Systems, Critical Analysis and Reasoning Skills (CARS), and the Psychological, Social, and Biological Foundations of Behavior. There are approximately 230 questions on the exam. Some call the MCAT the "Great Equalizer," as it can be tough to compare academic performance across hundreds of universities. Given differences in the competitiveness of institutions and grading methods, the MCAT enables admissions committees to compare students from different colleges to each other.

Though some argue that the test has no clear bearing on whether someone will be a good physician, several studies describe a relationship between the MCAT and academic performance in medical school. Thus, this test is not going anywhere. Moreover, on your journey to becoming a physician you will have to take many exams: first the MCAT, then the United States Medical Licensing Exam (USMLE) series (this consists of Step 1, Step 2 CK, Step 2 CS, and Step 3), then national subject-based examinations commonly referred to as shelf exams, and then finally your board certification examinations. For some specialties, board certification exams must be completed every five to ten years. I think it's fair to say that with time you will become a professional test taker! Medical schools and state licensing boards will continue to use these exams to determine your ability to practice medicine. Look at the MCAT as your official starting point. Develop good test-taking habits now, because you will most certainly need them as you work to become a physician.

The key to success in taking any test is to actually know and understand what is being tested. Visit the AAMC website for more information about the format of the MCAT exam. Purchase the AAMC's *Official Guide to the MCAT Exam*.[7] Become familiar with how the test is organized, the number of questions in each section, and understand how the examination is scored. The AAMC guide also provides tips on how to prepare, as well as over one hundred practice questions.

Next, you need to make sure that you commit enough time to study for the MCAT. If you know that you are someone who struggles with standardized testing (for example, you had difficulty with your ACT or SAT), then you may need a longer period of time to study compared to someone who may not have such difficulties. The phrase "know thy self" rings true here. Most people will attempt to take the MCAT exam during the second semester of their junior year. If you fall into this category, make sure that your course schedule will allow you to devote enough time to studying for the exam. If you are still taking classes while you are studying, be sure to avoid any courses that may be incredibly difficult or time-consuming during this time. You must be deliberate in committing yourself to the time and effort you need to succeed.

One of the biggest mistakes that students make when preparing for the MCAT is not taking enough practice exams. I recommend that students take a practice exam once a week, and do so every week until it is time for their MCAT. Try to take at least eight practice exams before taking the real thing. When you take your practice test, you should do everything you can to actually replicate test exam conditions. This means that you start with getting a good night's rest the night before, you take the exam at the same time in the morning every time, take breaks in the same manner that you would on the actual test day, wear what you would wear on test day, and eat on schedule the same way that you would if you were in the testing room. Do this once a week every week until your exam, and it will help you to develop the habits that you need to optimize your test-taking experience. By the time you get to your test, you should feel much less anxious about the process because you have been working under those same test conditions every week for the last eight to ten weeks. Purchase practice tests from any of the test prep companies, and be sure to purchase the practice tests made by the AAMC as well. Do the practice tests from the testing company first, and then, as you approach the test itself, complete practice tests from the AAMC. I recommend this order because you want to establish your knowledge base with the material first, and then really work on your test-taking skills using questions from the people who actually make the test.

With that said, do not take any practice tests less than one week before your actual exam. Nothing good can come from doing this. The odds are that you will psych yourself out and will make silly mistakes. Also, if you perform poorly on the practice and score lower than your goal, this will most certainly impact your confidence. Confidence is essential when you are preparing to take any standardized examination.

When you get questions wrong, force yourself to actually go back and understand the reason why you missed the question and what the concept is that you need to understand. This is so important! I often see students simply glance over the answers they got wrong without taking the time to actually understand the rationale behind *why* they chose the wrong answer and how to not make that mistake again. I would recommend you even go as far as creating either flashcards or some form of a table or chart where you outline all of the answers that you have gotten incorrect. This will allow you to go back and study those same concepts again to help reinforce them for the future. For concepts you can't seem to get, Google is your friend. You can easily search online for videos or special tutorials that will cover the concepts that you are struggling to understand. Chances are, if you're having trouble with the concept, there are thousands of other students who probably have that exact same question. Also, consider reaching out to your former teaching assistants from your pre-med classes. This is why it's always good to get to know your teaching assistants and professors really well (re-read the section on going to class every day), because more times than not they will be willing to help you get through a few challenging questions.

Finally—and this is a super important tip—plan on taking the MCAT only once! So many students make the mistake of taking the MCAT "just to see" how they will do. This is a big mistake. Every time you take a standardized test and do not perform well you undermine your confidence, which makes it harder to perform well on subsequent administrations of the test. Moreover, with each MCAT test that you take (and don't do well on), you call into question your academic ability and competence; the admissions committee will have to start wondering if you are able to handle the rigor of medical school. It is much better to delay your exam (yes, even if it means taking another year off) if it means that you are better prepared and will be able to take the test only once.

For some students reading this guide, your pre-med journey may already be well underway and may not have gone quite as planned. Perhaps you have not received good grades in some of the required pre-med classes, or have struggled on the MCAT. Do not give up on your dream just yet—you still have a chance to improve your application and make yourself a standout applicant. Over the last twenty years, more and more students are opting to take time off after their final year of college and before starting medical school. Known as a "gap year," some students choose to wait a year (or two or three!) before applying. This time can be used to complete a post-baccalaureate (post-bac) or special master's program to take coursework that will help to raise the BCPM GPA. These programs are also pursued by students who did not complete the pre-med prerequisites for some reason (stopped being pre-med, started the process late, or are a non-traditional applicant). You can find a pretty comprehensive list of these programs on the AAMC website. Some programs offer a master's degree or special certificate when the program is completed.

KEEP IT REAL DR. TOKS:

Should I get an MPH before going to medical school?

Being healthy is more than just the absence of disease, and pursuing an MPH (Master of Public Health) degree is an excellent way to broaden your understanding of health in our society, using public policy, epidemiology, and social science principles. I received an MPH degree while a medical student, and it has complimented my medical degree and helped to enhance my overall understanding of the healthcare system. While certainly an invaluable experience, many students pursue an MPH for the sole purpose of improving their chances

> to get accepted to medical school. Let's be clear—most of the courses in the MPH program WILL NOT boost your BCPM GPA. If that is what you are looking for, a post-bac or special master's program is the way to go. Do not fall for the hype—getting an MPH degree will not make a big difference in medical school admissions. Quite frankly, most admissions officers can see through these ulterior motivations. If you are truly interested in an MPH, some argue that it is best to pursue this either while you are a medical student or, even better (and much cheaper), through special fellowship/training programs during and after residency.

Still, some people choose to take a gap year for other reasons. At my medical school, about half of the incoming students took time off before matriculating. I chose to take two years off due to an illness in my family—and, quite frankly, I really needed a break! In my time off, I worked for an executive search firm—not remotely medical—and spent the rest of my time working with a nonprofit group that helped children with congenital birth defects. The decision to take time off is truly up to you. If you do decide to take a gap year, here are a few final things to keep in mind:

1. **Be deliberate.** Create a plan and be ready to explain the rationale for taking this time off. I know students

who took a year off because "it was the thing to do" and just moved around from job to job without any clear plan. Some students also try to complete a hundred different activities during this time, hoping that it will help their chances of admission. Often, the opposite is true; applicants can appear to lack focus and commitment when they become involved in too many activities.

2. **Make a significant impact.** Strive to make a difference in whatever you plan to do. For example, if you are really passionate about scientific research (and want to attend a medical school with a strong research emphasis), it may be helpful to pursue these research interests in your time off—and then aim to make a significant impact by producing a publication. Building on your interests is a great way to show the admissions committee your strengths.

3. **It does not always have to be an academic or "serious" endeavor.** In the right context, you can use your time off to do something that is personally rewarding and meaningful, or even a little outside the box. If you want to climb every mountain in North America, write your own book, or compete in extreme sports— you can use your time off for these activities. Presented in the right way, this will show the admissions committee the human aspect of your application, and will

certainly make for good conversation during the interview process! The path to a medical degree is long and grueling, so taking time off to pursue these sorts of activities can certainly be beneficial to mentally and emotionally recharge.

I personally recommend the 1 + 1 rule: Choose one endeavor that addresses either a major weakness in your application or builds upon a strength or interest, and then choose one "mini" activity that you consider really cool or interesting. For example: complete a post-bac program to help raise your GPA, while also taking hip-hop classes once a week because you have always loved dancing and now have some time to commit to this passion.

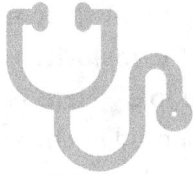

COMMITMENT TO MEDICINE

His booming voice transcended the thin walls, overpowering the usual hum of the small, working-class neighborhood. Seated in the crowded church, I listened closely as the reverend spoke about the curative power of prayer. At the close of his sermon, throngs of people rushed toward the pastor to receive a healing touch. I was both intrigued and dismayed by the great mass of people: I was fascinated by the pastor's ability to comfort the sick, yet troubled because many of the ailments for which the parishioners sought healing were preventable conditions—namely high cholesterol and hypertension. I realized then—though only a teenager—that serving as a physician would be my own way of alleviating the burden of disease in my community. Becoming a doctor was my calling.

*

When you ask students about their motivations for wanting to become a physician, the majority will simply answer: "Because I want to help people." Here is a not-so-secret secret: wanting to help people should *not* be your sole justification for becoming a doctor. While becoming a physician remains the greatest honor of my life, it has not come without significant stress, pain, and, quite frankly, financial investment. There are many other professions that can provide opportunities to help others without requiring the same level of personal sacrifice. So really think to yourself: why do I want to become a doctor?

Let's take a moment here to discuss some of the other reasons why you **should not** enter medicine. Despite what you may see on television, medical practice is not nearly as glamorous as it looks. While you may be mesmerized by Dr. House and his ability to diagnose the most obscure conditions, the reality is that as a physician, most of what you see will be "bread and butter" medicine—the most common conditions for which patients seek medical attention. As a pediatrician, I can spend the majority of my day performing routine physical exams for school athletic teams and treating ear infections. Now, don't get me wrong—I love this, but it is certainly a far cry from the excitement that you see on your favorite medical drama. When considering a career in medicine, be sure that you have an understanding of (1) what a *good* day looks like, (2) what a *bad* day looks like, and (3) what *most* days look like.

Students also commonly choose to pursue a medical career to satisfy their parents. Their parents may have always dreamed of having a doctor in the family, or they might want their child to follow in the footsteps of another physician in the family with a "stable" and "prestigious" career. But if you're only pursuing medicine as a means to make someone else happy, you may make a grave mistake. Seeking (and even obtaining) the approval of others may not be sufficient to overcome the challenges and costs of pursuing medicine. Again—I cannot emphasize this enough—there are many other ways to help others and make a difference in society. That's why it's so crucial to make sure that becoming a doctor is something that you really want to do.

I have also had students tell me that becoming a doctor is their "back-up" plan. Insert quizzical look here. As we have already discussed, becoming a physician takes an incredible amount of planning (as in, years in advance), and once you're in, YOU. ARE. IN. Something that takes so much time and effort to prepare for should not be a back-up plan. Don't forget, medical school is expensive, with the median education debt rising to $190,000 in 2016.[8] A back-up plan should not put you in this much debt! If you are considering another career and could see yourself doing something else besides being a doctor (and you would be happy with that other profession), I would strongly advise you to choose the other profession. When you have to go to the hospital at four in the morning in the middle of a snowstorm to take care of sick patients, only the love of medicine will sustain you. Trust me.

Before starting the process, I advise students to have an honest conversation with their parents and loved ones about what it takes to become a doctor. Many people are enamored by the image of doctors, but do not have a great understanding of what it takes to become a physician. These conversations are important, because as the road gets tough you will need the support of your friends and loved ones to help you through challenging times.

Now, with that out of the way, if after careful consideration you truly want to become a physician, let nothing stand in your way. Not age, not social situation, not race, not gender—nothing should stop you from pursuing your dream of becoming a doctor. Wearing that white coat is worth it. I am fortunate to know many physicians who did not take the traditional path to become a doctor, including a former lawyer, a nun, and a woman who was already a grandmother by the time she began medical school! If you want this career, you can make it happen.

Once you decide to become a physician, you must demonstrate your commitment to the medical field. The admissions committees want to see that you have made great efforts to better understand what it means to be a doctor and what working in our complex healthcare system entails. Ideally, you can show this commitment and effort through shadowing opportunities in medical settings. However, many students struggle with finding the right experiences. Shadowing can often feel like a passive activity. I can remember shadowing in a community clinic during my college years and feeling completely useless as I struggled to follow behind the doctor while she quickly moved between patient rooms. Your goal for shadowing should go beyond simply following the doctor around; you should strive to have a meaningful experience that will deepen your understanding and appreciation of medicine. Let's review a few important tips to make the most of your shadowing experience.

1. **Carefully select the doctor(s) who you shadow.** As you contemplate your career in medicine, you want to shadow a doctor in a specialty that most closely aligns with your interest. Take care in choosing who to shadow, because you should attempt to shadow this same person longitudinally, ideally over the course of several years. This will give you the chance not only to develop a strong relationship with the doctor (and perhaps get a letter of recommendation later on), but also the potential ability to see the same patients repeatedly, which can provide great insights about patient care and medical practice today. These interactions can also create interesting stories and become essay subjects when it comes time to write your personal statement. Here is a quick list of ways to find doctors that you can shadow:

- Check with your own primary care doctor
- Ask other doctors that you may know
- Talk with your pre-med advising office, which may have a list of doctors in the area willing to have students shadow
- Check your local hospital for volunteer programs
- Check your college's alumni directory—depending on the quality of the directory, you can usually do a search by profession and geography
- Do a simple online Google search to look for local physicians

Once you find a physician, how should you ask someone if you can shadow them? Given our digital age, I would suggest sending an email. Start your email off by introducing yourself. Mention your interest in medicine, and then discuss your interest in the doctor's particular specialty. Discuss why you're interested in their specialty and disclose any prior activities that you have done that support this interest. Flattery never hurts, so if you see that the doctor has great reviews online or was featured in a "Top Doctor" list, then mention that. Once you have sent your introductory email, if you do not hear back from the doctor within seventy-two hours, place a phone call to the office. **Do not** ask for the doctor to be pulled away from his or her clinical work to speak to you; leave a message with the secretary. Doctors are incredibly busy, so if the doctor does not get back to you or eventually declines your request, please don't take it personally.

2. **Dress the part.** You must dress formally, at least business casual. I generally prefer that men wear dress pants with a tie, and that women similarly dress in pants or a long skirt. Additionally, because you are in a medical setting, be sure to wear closed-toe shoes. And above all else, DO NOT wear a white coat! I had a student that did this once and it did not come across well. Wearing a white coat is a special honor (hence the white coat ceremony once you get to medical school), and donning a white coat while shadowing will give the impression that you are playing dress-up or are just plain obnoxious.

3. **Shadow for the whole job.** A physician's job extends beyond the day-to-day clinical duties. It also includes sitting in on committee and staff meetings, attending conferences, and sometimes developing research. Therefore, you should seek to experience the full scope of the job, not just seeing patients.

4. **Figure out how you can contribute to your doctor's work.** Did she forget the dose of amoxicillin? Look it up on the Epocrates app. Is the doctor running behind

schedule? Talk to patients that are waiting and help manage their expectations. This is all part of working in healthcare, and doing such tasks will likely win you the favor of the person that you are shadowing as well.

5. **Journal.** Be sure to write about your experiences in a small journal. Focus on your emotions and how you felt. Think about what you learned. When you journal, ask yourself: after my time today, why do I still want to be a doctor? Keeping this journal will be helpful for you as you reflect on your reasons for becoming a physician and will provide great material later on when you write your personal statement.

6. **Be courteous.** This should go without saying, but while shadowing, treat *everyone* that you meet with courtesy and respect—including the front office staff, the medical assistants, and the janitorial workers. I have had students shadow me who acted nice to the medical staff but treated the cafeteria workers with disrespect. Needless to say, once we discovered this, the student lost future shadowing opportunities. When you have completed your shadowing experience, be sure to write a note of thanks to the doctor. You can use email, but if possible try to send a handwritten thank-you card. If your experience has gone particularly well, you should ask for a letter of recommendation.

INTELLECTUAL CURIOSITY

"Numbers do not die. Our people do."[9]

Seated among soaring stacks of old medical journals in the library basement, I stumbled upon this quote during my thesis research on hypertension and cardiovascular disease within the African-American community. The author, J.N. Gayles, Jr., vividly describes his frustration with the healthcare system in inner cities. Though disease disparities between blacks and whites have been recognized for decades, these imbalances continue to persist. My studies soon became much more than an effort to fulfill my graduation requirement in history. I used this research opportunity to investigate the social trajectory of disease and the possible implications for healthcare delivery to disadvantaged groups. I learned to take the "road less traveled" in my approach to any problem, asking the questions others may not ask and observing less-than-conspicuous trends. I knew that as a future physician, I wanted to similarly engage in research that would provide sustainable solutions for disease prevention and healthy lifestyles within underserved communities.

Are you excited at the thought of being in a molecular biology lab and working under the hood? Are you an expert when it comes to using the pipette, or do you like working with lab animals? If you enjoy basic science research, you are certainly fulfilling an important aspect of becoming a physician by demonstrating an intellectual interest in the world around you. If you don't enjoy basic science research, do not worry—I am not that person either! I remember as an undergraduate hearing from my friends that I absolutely had to have basic science research experience in order to get into medical school. I followed their advice and talked to my organic chemistry professor, who kindly offered me a position in his lab. I did the work and stayed many late nights in the lab, but I became bored very quickly. Truthfully, I really did not have any interest in basic science research. My true passion was in history, and I eventually learned how to combine this interest with my pursuit of medicine. You need to understand that when medical schools ask for research, it does not necessarily mean basic science laboratory research. The research can take many forms. Doing a research project on patient safety and hospital quality or completing a research project on healthcare disparities is just as important as being in the research lab. In fact, the increasing focus on care quality in medicine provides many opportunities to show your intellectual curiosity. For example, you can do a research project examining the efficacy of healthcare screenings in a population of homeless veterans. You can research vaccination programs and their usage in international settings. You can even look at ways to prevent readmission at a local hospital. Ideally, the research would be somewhat related to medicine or the sciences, but any topic that is meaningful and important to you will work. The options are endless.

As a doctor, you always have to ask questions about the world around you. This is the basis of any research: asking a question about what you observe and using your problem-solving and critical thinking skills to systematically develop an answer. As a student, the benefits of research abound. It will increase your knowledge and teach you how to read primary academic literature. You will learn to think creatively about how to solve a specific problem. It will also teach you to think independently. The ability to think independently cannot be overemphasized: a saying you will often hear on the hospital wards is to "trust, but verify." This essentially means that even though you may be provided with an answer, you must be ready to question its validity and confirm the details on your own. As a physician, I can't tell you how many times I have been told that a patient had one particular diagnosis, but upon my own investigation quickly found that the patient was actually suffering from an entirely different problem. This is why research is so important, because it forces us to ask probing questions and find our own answers.

A successful research experience begins with examining a topic or subject area in which you are genuinely interested. Nothing is worse than engaging in a research experience about which you are not passionate. You will almost certainly not do your best work, and this disinterest will likely show once it comes time to interview for medical school. Secondly, when considering a research experience, try to think about ways to show commitment to the interest on a long-term basis. Ideally you will stay involved in the experience for more than just a few weeks. Additionally, you should make sure that your research experience demonstrates a commitment to the rigors of medical investigation by selecting an experience that encompasses the principles of the scientific method: asking a question, forming a hypothesis, developing a plan to test your hypothesis, and communicating the results of this testing in a meaningful way.

Outside of research, letters of recommendation offer another way for you to demonstrate your intellectual curiosity. Letters of recommendation are required for application to medical school. To be frank, most recommendation letters are pretty mediocre. Certainly, the letter-writer will likely comment about class performance and the grade earned, but a

GREAT letter will go beyond that. A great letter will discuss your intellectual curiosity, your overwhelming fund of knowledge, and how you went beyond the call of duty. To get this caliber of recommendation letter, always ask for a STRONG letter of recommendation—the key word being STRONG. By asking for a strong letter of recommendation, you are sending a message that you are looking for a letter that will really speak well about you—not just say, "Helen was a good student in my class and got an A." You want a letter that says: "Helen excelled in my organic chemistry class, and I would rank her as one of the best students I have encountered in my career. She took an active interest in the subject and made insightful and meaningful contributions to the course." Your letter of recommendation must address three things: your standing in the class, your accomplishments, and your personal characteristics (i.e., communication, maturity, and, most importantly, your potential for medical practice). You should ALWAYS provide your recommender with the most recent copy of your resume. Additionally, I also advise my students to prepare a brief document for the recommenders that highlights your grades, your major accomplishments during the class, and your personal interests. Detail is everything here. By providing this information in an easy-to-read format, you make your recommender's job much easier and are thus more likely to get a great letter. When I applied to medical school, I received letters of recommendation from my organic chemistry professor, my molecular biology professor, my history of science mentor, and a local community leader. To this day, I am grateful for their willingness to write on my behalf and help me get into medical school!

> **KEEP IT REAL DR. TOKS:**
>
> *Should I get a "famous" person in medicine to write a letter of recommendation for me?*
>
> It is best to have a variety of letters with different perspectives to give the admissions committee an image of you as a total person. So, for example, in addition to two letters of recommendation from science professors, you can also get a letter of recommendation from a work supervisor, a coach, or someone who you have done community service with. Sometimes students make the mistake of obtaining a letter from a "prominent person" like a famous doctor, award-winning scientist, or renowned professor that they don't really know in hopes that this will impress the admissions committee. It probably won't. What you really want is someone who knows you well and can write about you in an exciting and meaningful way. On the flip side, do not ask for let-

> ters of recommendation from family members or close friends—the admissions officer almost certainly won't take such letters seriously and you will lose credibility, as they will likely consider these letters to be biased.

One last bit of advice here: always ask for a letter of recommendation as soon as possible. It is important to ask for the recommendation early because it may take your letter-writer much longer than expected to get the letter completed—and you want them to write a compelling and thoughtful letter on your behalf, right? Remember, awaiting recommendation letters can result in significant delays in processing the application package. Finally, one week before your personal deadline for the letter, remind your letter-writer of the due date if they have yet to get it to you.

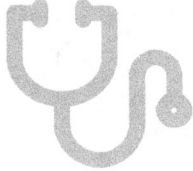

COMPASSION AND SERVICE

Born with Down's syndrome, RJ had become a familiar face in the hospital. At only seven months old, she awaited surgery to correct a cardiac anomaly, but had been admitted again for shortness of breath. She became one of my first pediatric patients as a medical student. The senior resident—believing that RJ's presentation was pretty simple—assigned RJ to me. I spent a lot of time with RJ and her mother. RJ needed special care requiring tremendous energy, and her mother felt especially burdened as she struggled to navigate the healthcare system as a non–English speaker. In our conversations, I soon discovered that her mother was less worried about her breathing and much more concerned about RJ's inability to move her right leg. I shared this information with my resident immediately. Skeletal radiologic surveys, bone scans, and many tough questions later, we found that RJ suffered abuse from the hands of a family member. My role quickly evolved from medical student to patient advocate.

My favorite medical quote is from Dr. William Osler, the father of modern medicine and one of the founding professors of Johns Hopkins Hospital: "Just listen to your patient; he is telling you the diagnosis."[10] At the core of being a physician is the ability to demonstrate compassion and empathy toward others. In the case of RJ, we almost missed an important diagnosis because we did not seek to fully understand the mother's concerns in the early hours of her presentation.

Being a good doctor requires more than ordering tests and prescribing medications. Your patient is much more than the disease or ailment with which they have been diagnosed—they actually have a life outside of their illness. One of the greatest medical professors that I ever encountered at Yale, Dr. Cyrus Kapadia, used to tell us to never use "male" or "female" in the opening sentence of our patient presentations on rounds—we had to say "gentleman" or "lady." His intention was to remind us that patients are not objects, but people. Your patients will need you to lend a compassionate ear as they struggle with fear, sadness, hopelessness, and despair. We often forget that the treatment plan that we give to patients includes showing respect for who they are and making sure they feel well-supported.

Admittedly, in our increasingly complex healthcare system, it may not always be easy to demonstrate compassion. Doctors are required to see more and more patients in a shorter period of time, and the demands of clinical paperwork are downright burdensome. Even in medical school, where it is expected that students can learn these skills, the anxiety of having to study constantly and perform well academically often causes medical students to prioritize the technical aspects of medicine. However, as a pre-medical student, you have the unique opportunity—and the time—to demonstrate and build on these humanistic qualities. My second favorite medical quote is often credited to Hippocrates: "cure sometimes, treat often, comfort always." You may not quite be at the point in your training where you can cure or treat, but it certainly does not take a medical degree to learn how to comfort. Use some of your extracurricular activities as a forum to cultivate this skill.

Generally speaking, your medical school application needs to demonstrate proficiency in three areas: patient exposure, academic engagement, and community service. We have already discussed shadowing and scholarly pursuits, so let's now take a moment to address service to others. Ideally, applicants will have at least 100–150 hours of community service before they apply to medical school. This may seem like a lot, but the key is to do these activities over the course of several years. You can serve your community in various ways—and they do not necessarily need to directly relate to healthcare. For example, as a pre-med student my service activities included developing a reading program at the local elementary school. Organizing relief efforts for natural disasters, mentoring disadvantaged children, volunteering for the Special Olympics—the opportunities for service are endless. All it takes is a genuine interest and commitment to others.

With that said, do not participate in activities because it is currently "in vogue" or the one thing you heard that all pre-meds must do. For example, many students will pursue international experiences because they think it will make them appear more impressive to the admissions committee. We all know the applicant who built water wells in Port-au-Prince during his gap year or the student who worked on HIV education initiatives in Bangladesh. While such endeavors are indeed meaningful, participation in these experiences often requires a significant financial investment that many students can't afford. Don't worry, you can still demonstrate your compassion for others without incurring such expenses. And quite frankly, admissions committees can see right through students who participate in these international experiences just for show.

KEEP IT REAL DR. TOKS:

How many extracurricular activities should I be involved in?

There is no "magic number" of extracurricular activities that students should be involved in.

However, every year I work with pre-medical students that have made the mistake of signing up for TOO many activities. The reality is that most of these activities have no meaningful or lasting significance for them. The key here is quality, not quantity. While participation in a one-time walkathon for diabetes or a donation to a blood drive is awesome, it is more important to participate in only a few activities that have been meaningful to you over the course of several years. Thus, in your initial years of college, really take the time to understand what issues are truly important to you and what you are passionate about. That way, you can use those interests to guide your future involvement in extracurricular activities. Now don't get me wrong, one-time extraordinary opportunities should not be missed; for example, a study abroad experience or participation in a summer science research program. But don't make the mistake of signing up for a bunch of different activities thinking that you will sound more impressive to the admissions committees. If anything, it will make you seem like you lack focus, and the admissions committee will know right away that you only seek to impress them. Also, you don't want all of these activities to take away from your studies!

One last note about your activities, don't be afraid to be different. This is the time to not only highlight your compassion and empathy, but also to show your personality and interests that may not come through in other parts of your application. For example, I know someone who loves breakdancing and spent a large chunk of his time dancing with children in a local group. I know of another medical school applicant who loves technology and spent his time creating a new software program to change the way that students study. It is okay to be unique—don't do certain activities just because you've heard about other people doing the same things.

Consider opportunities that will challenge your own preconceived notions and get you out of your comfort zone. As a doctor, you will have to take care of people who may hold a different set of beliefs than you, patients that may be considered to be "difficult," and people who society has repeatedly shunned and marginalized. Regardless of your personal values, these patients still have the right to be treated with respect and they deserve empathy. Working with teenagers in a juvenile detention facility or creating health materials for substance abusers are unique opportunities to advocate for your patient and demonstrate compassion to those who certainly need it.

Finally, remember that you will be required to document several details about your extracurricular activities when you apply to medical school by filling out an online form. Next to the personal statement, this is often considered to be the toughest part of the application. How can you make it easier? From the first day of college (or as soon as you decide to pursue medicine), keep a log of every activity in which you have participated. This should include the name of the activity, the supervisor, the number of hours that you spent participating, and when the activity was completed. You should also include your accomplishments, awards, and any other pertinent details about the activity. For activities that you really enjoyed or achieved great success, I encourage students to write a few sentences about the experience as it is happening. This will help you when it comes time to write the mini essay on your "most meaningful" activity for your medical school application.

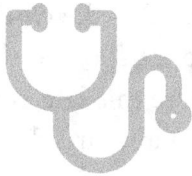

TEAMWORK AND COMMUNICATION

On a cold Friday night, our team learned that a kidney became available for transplantation. I was a third-year medical student rotating on transplant surgery. By 1:00am, I was sandwiched between five big, tall men in blue gowns in the South Pavillion operating suite. I stood next to a world-renowned surgeon, who was speaking excitedly to the other doctors in the room. As the new third-year medical student, I really did not understand what was going on and admittedly did not really enjoy surgical procedures. My only job for the night: retraction. I was asked to use the retractor tool to hold back the folds of skin so that the internal organs would be in clear view for the surgeons. Unfortunately, I am no night owl, and as the evening wore on my left arm grew tired from using the retractor. My thoughts drifted to my bed. Instead of looking at the surgical field, I gazed at the clock, hoping the surgeons would finish the procedure soon so that I could go to sleep. Why did I need to be here this late anyway, when there were five "real" doctors at the table already?

"Medical student, you are killing the kidney!"

I quickly snapped out of my sleepy thoughts. The retractor had come a little too close to the kidney. All eyes in the room were turned toward me. I had not paid attention to my one task, and my lack of focus almost caused injury to this organ—a **life-saving** kidney. Being on the spot like that all of a sudden makes you wake up, and I returned to my retracting job with laser-sharp focus—for the next several hours.

Every time I think of this story, I can't help but blush. I remember how scared I was when the surgeon turned his attention toward me, and how embarrassed I felt that I had temporarily failed my team. This brings me to the next important quality of being a great physician: teamwork. As a then-medical student, I tuned out because I didn't understand the significance of my role on the team. But one of the most important aspects of being a physician is the ability to work with other people and recognize that everyone on the medical team brings value to the table. Admittedly, I took this for granted as a student. When people stressed the importance of working with others, I dismissed such statements as tired clichés; after all, knowledge is the most important thing, right? But being a team player is critical as a physician. You cannot take care of patients alone. Good teamwork can truly make the difference between giving the patient excellent care and placing the patient at risk of a serious medical error.

To have a good team requires having good communication. Without quality communication, the work of the team becomes useless. The lack of clear direction leads to messages getting lost and priorities becoming misaligned. Let's take a brief moment to address a few of the critical aspects to good communication.

An important key to effective communication is to make sure that your message is clear. When you are dealing with very complex medical information, you don't want important details to get lost in translation. Because of this, it is essential that your message is clear, simple, and appropriately conveys urgent information. This is best exemplified during the daily "sign-out." The daily sign-out is a dedicated time in the hospital, typically in the morning and in the evening, when physicians come together. Whether you are leaving or just starting your shift, sign-out is where you communicate about the current patient census, important events, and critical next steps that need to happen in the patient's care. You would think that this would be a pretty straightforward process, but there is actually an art to giving a good sign-out. Don't say enough, and you may miss sharing important details about the patient.

Give too much detail, and the recipient will likely start to roll their eyes and not listen to all that you have to say! You have to be specific: why *exactly* do you want the only nighttime doctor in the whole hospital to spend precious time to check those labs? Having clear and simple messaging is truly an important skill.

Another frequently overlooked aspect of effective communication is knowing your audience. The way that I share information with a teenaged boy about his medical illness will likely differ from how I deliver a similar message to an elderly woman with early-stage dementia. Knowing your audience also means that you recognize the potential barriers and possible misconceptions that people may have in understanding your message. Education and literacy can be a major barrier: estimates show that just over 20 percent of adults read at the most basic reading level.[11] This statistic should encourage us to avoid medical jargon whenever possible and focus on keeping the message simple and clear. If the patient does not understand the message, they will not feel empowered to take the steps needed to safeguard their health. Knowing your audience also means knowing the background and cultural beliefs of your patients. I once had an elderly African-American man as a patient, and his wife often refused to let us run necessary tests because she was concerned that he would become a "guinea pig"—her beliefs were rooted in a distrust of the health system given our nation's history of discrimination towards people of color. This is why knowing your audience is so critical. Remember that, as a physician, your audience will include not only your patients and their families, but also other members of the care team. You will have to speak with administrators and talk to insurance companies. You will have to give presentations in front of groups, convince the on-call neurosurgeon to come into the hospital to see your patient at two in the morning, and share your research with your peers. It cannot be overstated that effective communication is at the heart of delivering quality medical care to patients.

KEEP IT REAL DR. TOKS:

What should I do about my weaknesses?

Sometimes being a good team player means communicating your weaknesses as well; looking back at that time in the operating room, perhaps I should have spoken up to the other doctors and shared that I was having difficulty. Some of you may scoff at revealing such vulnerability, but being honest in this way can have real, life-saving implications. For example, when a patient is dying and the team is performing chest compressions to save the patient's life, it is important that the chest compressions are done properly and with enough force.

> Unlike what you see on television, your arms can easily become tired. When this happens you have to speak up so that another member can step in and take your place—someone's life is at stake.
>
> With that said, everyone has weaknesses. No one is perfect in medicine. You don't have to bare your entire soul to the admissions committee, but it is okay to acknowledge shortcomings, such as a bad test score. Doctors are not infallible, and being honest about your weaknesses demonstrates humility and allows the admissions committee to see the "human" side of you.

From time to time you'll see doctors that will bark orders at nurses and ancillary staff, which oftentimes leads staff members to become afraid of engaging those doctors. In my career, I have witnessed numerous times where the nurse was worried that an order for a patient looked incorrect but did not speak up because she feared that the physician would yell and become upset. This brings me to perhaps the most important key to effective communication: good communication involves so much more than just talking. It also incorporates the ability to truly listen to what others have to say. Having the ability to listen well requires that you actually pay attention. Everyone has important information to contribute; I can't even begin to count the number of times that a nurse or a physical therapist reminded me of critical information that shaped a patient's care plan. Your patients want to know that you are listening too: when your patient sees that you are actually taking the time to listen to them, it often promotes greater trust and strengthens the patient-physician relationship. This can help you get to the root cause of the patient's problem, which in turn allows you to diagnose the patient much more quickly. The inability or unwillingness to listen to others is not only a matter of getting the message wrong; it may mean life or death for the patient in your care.

Being a great team player and a good communicator are lifelong skills that require continual practice. Start learning early—which is where your extracurricular activities again become important. We have already talked about the role of extracurricular activities, but now I want you to take it one step further by asking you to think about deliberately participating in opportunities that will give you the chance to build on your communication skills. Serving as a leader of a student group is a great way to demonstrate your ability to communicate effectively. Admissions committees are not looking for leadership experience simply because it makes you seem accomplished, but rather participating in leadership roles lets them know that you understand the value of teamwork and communication. As a leader, the very success of your group or organization will often lie in your ability to communicate well with others. You have to be able to connect with many different people and personalities. You have to be able to communicate the mission of your group so that others understand that mission and become invested in the success of the organization. Quite simply, you want to be able to inspire others to action. This is what admissions committees want.

So don't shy away from opportunities to take on leadership positions; such experiences are more than resume builders, they also provide you with a great opportunity to build your teamwork and communication skills. Achieving this will prove to yourself, and show to medical schools, that you have what it takes to become a great physician.

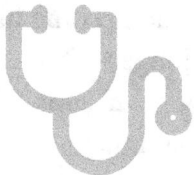

ETHICAL PRINCIPLES AND INTEGRITY

Despite living in the United States for over forty years, Mrs. Batiste still spoke with a soft French accent. Mrs. Batiste remained in the hospital bed—today was day eighty-six—and she could barely move. The body that once danced in local talent shows now appeared frail and tired. Metastatic pancreatic cancer ravaged her body—her skin pale, her eyes closed, and her lips dry. It was clear to the medical team that she would likely pass in a matter of weeks, maybe even in a few days. We had already treated her with every therapy available and exhausted all of our treatment options. Mrs. Batiste's two sons felt otherwise. Despite witnessing the fast decline of their mother, they still wanted the medical team to continue treatments that at this point had become futile. The current issue? Mrs. Batiste would no longer eat, a telltale sign of the early stages of death. However, her sons felt that if we were able to increase her nutritional intake, she would be able to eventually improve enough to tolerate another round of chemotherapy. They requested that the medical team put a feeding tube in place. While a tube in this case could offer the benefit of nourishment, it would likely be only temporary. Feeding tubes are also very uncomfortable and carry a risk of aspiration. These risks were explained to the patient's family, but they still wanted to move forward with placing the tube. After much discussion, the case was moved to the hospital ethics committee.

Ethical dilemmas in medicine happen all of the time. People most commonly think of abortion, euthanasia, and stem cell research as the most often-encountered ethical dilemmas, but the case of Mrs. Batiste is in no way unique. As a medical student, I underestimated the degree to which I would soon have to make very tough decisions as a future physician. What do you do when a parent of a child refuses blood transfusions because of their religious faith? How do you manage a situation where the estranged wife and the live-in girlfriend both show up at a dying man's bedside? How do you handle a case where a patient who is newly infected with HIV demands that you not share this information with her husband? These are all very real issues that you may encounter as a physician, so it is important that you know how to approach such problems. When you interview for a medical school, you will be asked for your perspective on an important ethical issue or a moral dilemma. It can be tough to make these decisions. Where should you begin?

First, take some time to really consider your own position on several important ethical issues in medicine. I have listed below a non-exhaustive list of the most common questions that should serve as a pretty solid launching point.

- If you are not working clinically, should you assist a person in medical distress?
- Can a parent refuse treatment for their child?
- What do you do if your patient refuses treatment?
- How do you feel about abortion?
- Should you ever withhold information from a patient?
- And, as in the story above, would you give a treatment to a patient that you know is futile?

When thinking about these dilemmas, do not focus on giving an answer that you think people want to hear. Start with acknowledging any legal considerations (for example, as seen with abortion). Then try to consider both sides of the argument and the pros and cons for either side. Finally, when coming to an answer, you must consider the four key principles of medical ethics: patient autonomy, justice, beneficence, and non-maleficence. Here is a quick overview:

Autonomy: Does my response respect the patient's right to make their own decisions?

Beneficence: Does my response consider the benefits to the patient?

Non-maleficence: Does my response lead to or cause the patient harm in any way?

Justice: Does my response have broader implications going beyond the patient and into the community at large?

The goal of this framework is to put the patient at the center of ethical decision-making. Sometimes, the principles may be in tension with one another (for example, a patient may have the right to make their own decision but the decision may cause significant harm). While you may not come up with a single best answer, it is up to you as the provider to be sensitive to the nuances and multi-dimensionality of the issues presented by these ethical quandaries. A good book to read on medical ethics is *Clinical Ethics: A Practical Approach to Ethical Decisions in Clinical Medicine.*[12] Use this guide, and you should be well on your way.

> ## KEEP IT REAL DR. TOKS:
>
> ### *When applying to medical school, what do I need to know about health insurance?*
>
> Be sure to know about the Affordable Care Act and the fundamental ethical issues behind it—including whether access to healthcare is a fundamental human right. You do not necessarily need to understand every single detail of the law, but you should certainly understand the basic premise of its creation, its impact on the medical field thus far, and the reasons why people agree with or object to the legislation. Physicians need to remain aware of current events in medicine, so you should be able to show the admissions committee that you have this understanding.

In addition to ethical principles, at the core of being a physician is integrity. The Oxford dictionary defines integrity as "the quality of being honest and having strong moral principles."[13] I like another definition: doing the right thing when no one else is watching you.[14] It is this integrity that is critical to the patient-physician relationship and therefore carries great weight. Being a doctor comes with a lot of responsibility, first to the patient, but also to insurance agencies, state and federal government bodies, and, yes, even to public companies. For example, nearly every primary care doctor can share stories where patients have asked to have a note for an employer providing the patient with a leave of absence from work. Some patients try to push the limit on this. I once had a patient ask me to list his return to work date as a week later so that he could spend some extra time with his family at home. Seems innocent enough (and who wouldn't want to spend more time with family?), but as a physician you have a duty to report only on the medical necessity of the patient's absence from work. And the reality is that work absences cost billions of dollars a year; a 2015 report from the Centers for Disease Control Foundation suggests that absenteeism costs employers well over $200 billion annually.[15] As a doctor, your medical opinion can impact high profile court decisions, determine whether a person can receive disability, and influence a utility provider's decision to continue providing electricity to a home despite the family's inability to pay. It also means that you do not let personal benefit or monetary gain impact your decision-making; many medical schools ban pharmaceutical companies from giving talks to students, and it is standard that a physician discloses financial relationships or special interests before giving professional talks. Physicians are indeed held to a higher standard.

So, as a pre-med student how can you demonstrate integrity? The most obvious way would be through your recommendation letters. Your recommenders should be the people that know you best, who can attest to the quality of your character and can speak on this very topic. This is why it is critical that the people writing your letters of recommendation know you very well and can comment on these personal qualities. (And to be clear, hopefully you are doing the right thing because it is the right thing to do, not just to be seen).

Your personal statement offers another important opportunity to highlight examples of integrity. While grades and test scores may indeed be at the forefront of your evaluation by medical schools, a high-quality personal statement can truly make the difference between an acceptance and a rejection. Many students make the mistake of rehashing details of their academic performance or extracurricular activities in the personal statement, but this is your chance to not only state your interest in medicine, but also to show how you possess the essential qualities—like integrity—needed to become a good physician. The key word here is "show." Don't just say in your personal essay that you have integrity, you want to describe a situation and demonstrate how you have shown this quality. You can do this by writing a clear, vivid, engaging, and compelling narrative. The best essays will also include very personal and honest reflections on some of the challenges of being a physician.

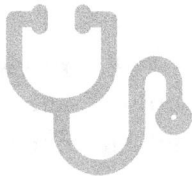

PROFESSIONALISM

I woke up late, again, and barely had enough time to see my assigned patient on the Fitkin Medical Service that morning. I was on my internal medicine rotation as a fourth-year medical student and I was expected to know everything about the two patients assigned to me. Every morning at 7:30 a.m. we started our rounds, and it was my job to present the patient in front of the attending and the residents on the team. Because it was my last week on the rotation, my attending made clear to me that he preferred that I not read from my notes when presenting; adjusting his royal blue bow tie he would say to me—"This is YOUR patient. Tell me what you know." I had gotten away with still using my notes for the last several days, but of course today was going to be different. Unfortunately, I spent the night before catching up with old friends and simply lost track of time—8:00 p.m. soon turned into 3:00 a.m. I had meant to iron my slacks that morning but had to run out the door in order to get to the hospital. My short white coat had red and black pen marks from my multicolored pen. I looked a mess. I started to present my patient, looking down at my notes as usual, and was quickly interrupted.

"From memory, Dr. Famakinwa. This is YOUR patient."

I couldn't believe it. I placed my notes down on the computer next to me, cleared my throat, and began the presentation. After repeating the patient's name and chief complaint, I drew a blank, and could not remember any of the patient details that I had scribbled down on my notes only minutes before. As I attempted to formulate an assessment and plan for the patient's care, I completely stumbled. The cold stares from my resident and the attending confirmed my complete flop. Not my finest moment.

My attending then asked the senior resident to present the patient. In his crisp white coat, he stepped into the center of the circle and flawlessly presented the details of the patient's presentation, overnight events, and upcoming plans for the day. He then did this for every single patient on the service. Without notes. I was completely embarrassed. I learned my lesson: always come prepared, always come on time, and at the very least, look the part.

*

The American Board of Medical Specialties defines medical professionalism as "a belief system in which group members ('professionals') declare ('profess') to each other and the public the shared competency standards and ethical values they promise to uphold in their work and what the public and individual patients can and should expect from medical professionals."[16] Professionalism goes beyond a code of conduct manual filled with rules and regulations. Quite simply, professionalism is the way in which we inspire confidence. Patients should feel confident in the care that you provide; similarly, your colleagues need to have confidence in your ability as well. We have already addressed some of the ethical and moral aspects of professionalism, and now we will shift to a few other key principles to keep in mind. Some of these things may seem like common knowledge, but as the saying goes, "common knowledge is not always common."

1. **Taking responsibility.** As a physician, you are responsible for the most precious of all things—another human life. This responsibility obligates you to provide the best care to your patient possible. This may mean that you have to stay a little longer at work to ensure that your patient receives proper care. You may need to stay awake an hour longer to read an article about available treatments for an obscure disease. To be sure, sometimes taking responsibility is not easy—I remember a few times as an intern having to admit to the senior medical attending that I did not look up a

critical piece of information about a patient. Embarrassing, yes, but far more embarrassing is what I have seen others do, which is to avoid taking responsibility for their actions and to lie—this just never goes well.

2. **Physical Presentation.** Many people underestimate just how conservative the practice of medicine is. I would never tell someone to hide who they are or to suppress their need for self-expression, but it is important to keep in mind your audience. You do not want to wear things that may alienate your patients or colleagues in any way. How do you put this in practice now? As tempting as it may be otherwise, try to dress properly for class and avoid going in your pajamas (seriously, I hear this is becoming a trend). I know that this may be difficult, and, as my college friends will tell you, I loved wearing baggy sweatpants with matching bandanas in my early years. However, the goal is to be professional and put your best foot forward. I once worked with a student who wore suits to class every day during our summer program. Because he looked professional, all of the professors took notice and viewed him favorably. His appearance conveyed maturity and seriousness about his medical pursuits. This actually opened the door for him to receive additional opportunities that the other students just didn't get. Now, I am not saying that you need to wear a three-piece suit to school every day, but certainly dressing your best

matters. Remember, while it is tough to wake up and get dressed in time for that 7:00 a.m. class, there will come a day when you will be expected to be at the hospital dressed professionally and seeing patients at 5:00 a.m. So get in the habit now!

3. **Punctuality.** If you are five minutes early, you're on time, and if you are on time you are late. Being punctual does not only apply to seeing patients in a timely fashion, it also extends to completing the paperwork on time as well. This is critical for legal reasons. It is also important because there are other physicians that are likely depending on your paperwork as they strive to provide care for your patient as well. If you constantly turn in work late, consider working on your time management and organization skills so that this does not become a problem in the long run.

4. **Trustworthiness.** Personally, the most humbling aspect of being a physician is that patients are trusting me with the most intimate and personal details of their lives. For patients to share these details they must feel as if they can trust their doctor. Once upon a time, physicians were given carte blanche in their care for patients. However, given recent reports on the increasing number of medical errors and a shameful history of inappropriate treatment of marginalized groups in our society, patients have become increas-

ingly wary and skeptical of the healthcare system. This mistrust interferes with quality care; if the patient does not trust you, they may omit critical information necessary for determining their actual diagnosis. Furthermore, because of the sensitive nature of health information, patients have to trust that these details will not be inappropriately shared with others.

CONCLUSION

February is often considered to be one of the most difficult months of the year as a resident. In many parts of the country (especially Connecticut), cold weather and winter storms abound. You never get to see the sun; when you leave for work it is dark outside, and when you return home, it is dark once again. The patient census is much higher, and longer hours in the hospital mean less time spent with family and loved ones.

February 2015 was no exception, especially as I was going through a rough time in my own life. My car slid on ice and hit a divider as I returned home from a night shift. I was the senior on the oncology unit, and our service was at capacity with very ill patients. As I was completing two residencies in one, I had less clinical experience on the wards than my colleagues in the traditional residency programs, which caused me to second-guess my medical decisions. I just did not feel like a competent doctor. It also didn't help that Mrs. Franco was assigned to my team. Recently diagnosed with lung cancer, she had gained notoriety throughout the hospital for being a difficult and demanding patient. Her drinking water had to be ice-cold, she would not let the medical team see her until after eleven, and she frequently argued with the physicians about her treatment plan. One evening, I had managed to wrap up my work a little early and planned to go home. However, we always had a particularly tough time with Mrs. Franco during morning rounds, so I figured I should go to her room a second time and update her on the goals for the next day. As I took a deep breath and began to tell her the plan, she stopped me mid-sentence:

"You know, I have to tell you, you are really a great doctor. I wish you had your own office outside the hospital—I would definitely come to you. I can tell, being a doctor is truly your gift in life. You are fulfilling your life's purpose."

Right there, in front of Mrs. Franco, my patient, I broke down crying. To hear her say those words to me, after I had been questioning the direction of my own life and my value as a new doctor, meant everything to me. It was exactly what I needed to hear to keep me going.

As a physician, you will soon see that patients enrich our lives just as much as we seek to provide care to save theirs. This is the true beauty of the patient-physician relationship. Even on the hardest of days, I am grateful that I have a career that allows me to connect deeply with people, alleviate human suffering, and restore health. As an attending physician now, I still continue to learn and grow each and every day. This is what makes medicine exciting! I can't believe that I began this journey in medicine almost two decades ago, but I have no regrets and would not change my experiences for anything.

I know that it is easy to get lost in the statistics and numbers. As you continue your day-to-day pre-med grind, I hope that this book will not only provide you with helpful admissions advice, but also remind you of why being a physician is truly an honor.

So roll up your sleeves, grab your computer, and get to work. You got this!

REFERENCES

1. "Table A-7: Applicants, First-Time Applicants, Acceptees, and Matriculants to U.S. Medical Schools by Sex, 2008-2009 through 2017-2018." Association of American Medical Colleges. Accessed September 24, 2018. https://www.aamc.org/download/321470/data/factstablea7.pdf.

2. "Table A-16: MCAT Scores and GPAs for Applicants and Matriculants to U.S. Medical Schools, 2016-2017 through 2017-2018." Association of American Medical Colleges. Accessed September 24, 2018. https://www.aamc.org/download/321494/data/factstablea16.pdf.

3. "Mission." Accessed September 24, 2018. http://www.med.unc.edu/www/about/about-the-school-of-medicine-1/mission.

4. "About | University of Pittsburgh School of Medicine." University of Pittsburgh School of Medicine. Accessed September 24, 2018. https://www.medschool.pitt.edu/about.

5. "Mission | Yale School of Medicine." Accessed September 24, 2018. https://medicine.yale.edu/about/mission.aspx.

6. "Table A-17: MCAT Scores and GPAs for Applicants and Matriculants to U.S. Medical Schools by Primary Undergraduate Major, 2017-2018." Association of American Medical Colleges. Accessed September 24, 2018. https://www.aamc.org/download/321496/data/factstablea17.pdf

7. The "Official Guide to the MCAT Exam" can be purchased at https://members.aamc.org.

8. Brin, Dinah Wisenberg. "Taking the Sting Out of Medical School Debt." AAMC News. April 04, 2017. Accessed September 24, 2018. https://news.aamc.org/medical-education/article/taking-sting-out-medical-school-debt/.

9. Gayles, J.N. "Health Brutality and the Black Life Cycle." Black Scholar 5 (May 1974): 2- 9.

10. Gandhi, Jadeep Singh. "Re: William Osler: A Life in Medicine." The BMJ. Accessed September 24, 2018. https://www.bmj.com/content/321/7268/1087.2/rr/760724. Originally published: BMJ 2000;321:1087.

11. Safeer, Richard S., and Jann Keenan. "Health Literacy: The Gap Between Physicians and Patients." American Family Physician 72, no. 3 (2005): 463-68. Accessed online September 24, 2018.

12. Jonsen, Albert R., William J. Winslade, and Mark Siegler. Clinical Ethics: A Practical Approach to Ethical Decisions in Clinical Medicine. New York: McGraw-Hill, 2015.

13. "Integrity | Definition of Integrity in English by Oxford Dictionaries." Oxford Dictionaries | English. Accessed September 24, 2018. https://en.oxforddictionaries.com/definition/integrity.

14. This quote is often misattributed to C.S. Lewis, when in fact the origin is reportedly a paraphrase of a statement made by Charles Marshall. See Living the Legacy of C.S. Lewis. http://www.cslewis.org/aboutus/faq/quotes-misattributed/. Accessed September 24, 2018.

15. "Worker Illness and Injury Costs U.S. Employers $225.8 Billion Annually." CDC Foundation. January 28, 2015. Accessed September 24, 2018. https://www.cdcfoundation.org/pr/2015/worker-illness-and-injury-costs-us-employers-225-billion-annually.

16. American Board of Medical Specialties. ABMS Definition of Medical Professionalism (Long Form). Chicago, IL, 2012. Developed by the Ethics and Professionalism Committee-ABMS Professionalism Work Group.

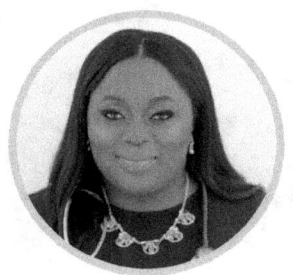

ABOUT THE AUTHOR

Dr. Olatokunbo Famakinwa, better known as Dr. Toks, is an award-winning physician who is board certified in both pediatrics and internal medicine. Among her other accolades, she was most recently presented with the American Medical Association's Excellence in Medicine Leadership Award. She is a graduate of the Yale School of Medicine and additionally earned a master's in public health from Harvard University.

Dr. Toks has always been determined to alleviate the burden of preventable disease in all communities, large and small. Drawing on her experiences, she is also committed to supporting a new generation of medical professionals from within these communities. A child of Nigerian immigrants, Dr. Toks enjoys African dance, reading, and spending time with family. She lives in Washington, DC.

To learn more, visit her website at www.doctortoksmd.com

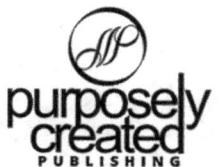

CREATING DISTINCTIVE BOOKS
WITH INTENTIONAL RESULTS

We're a collaborative group of creative masterminds with a mission to produce high-quality books to position you for monumental success in the marketplace.

Our professional team of writers, editors, designers, and marketing strategists work closely together to ensure that every detail of your book is a clear representation of the message in your writing.

Want to know more?
Write to us at info@publishyourgift.com
or call (888) 949-6228

Discover great books, exclusive offers, and more at
www.PublishYourGift.com

Connect with us on social media

@publishyourgift

www.ingramcontent.com/pod-product-compliance
Lightning Source LLC
Chambersburg PA
CBHW052203110526
44591CB00012B/2053